Massage for Two:

All the Secrets From A to Z, the Use of Essential Oils and More

I0429187

Fill Sunrik

Massage for Two

CONTENTS

Chapter 1

Massage for Two: What Is It?

Erotic massage - a wonderful craft that can be discussed for hours, but it is better to master it and enjoy it. It's an extraordinary tool with which you can present yourself in the eyes of the person you are in love with. No wonder women in the East have perfectly mastered this craft, having absorbed it in their mother's milk in early childhood. As a result, their husbands are always satisfied and are in good spirits.

Erotic massage is a wonderful relaxation technique, known since time immemorial, and is also a great way to create a strong bond between lovers. With massage, it is easy to show care and trust, which are necessary in love. A joint sexual massage, which strongly stimulates is an unsurpassed way to learn about the desires and feelings of a loved one. Like dancing, a good massage takes two. It is wonderful if, during the massage, the partners fully approve each other's actions with the help of groans or sighs. So they develop their own language of gestures and sounds, understandable only to them. To relieve fatigue and bring the body into a state of comfort and harmony, massage is used during sexual foreplay. An erotic massage is no place for embarrassment. Erotic massages (intimate massages) are the key to the development of sexuality and sensitivity. This type of massage is done in the nude, with the purpose of sexual stimulation, it is no secret that sexual arousal occurs when you touch the erogenous zones. Remarkably, your love games are always preceded by a mutual massage session.

Massage for Two

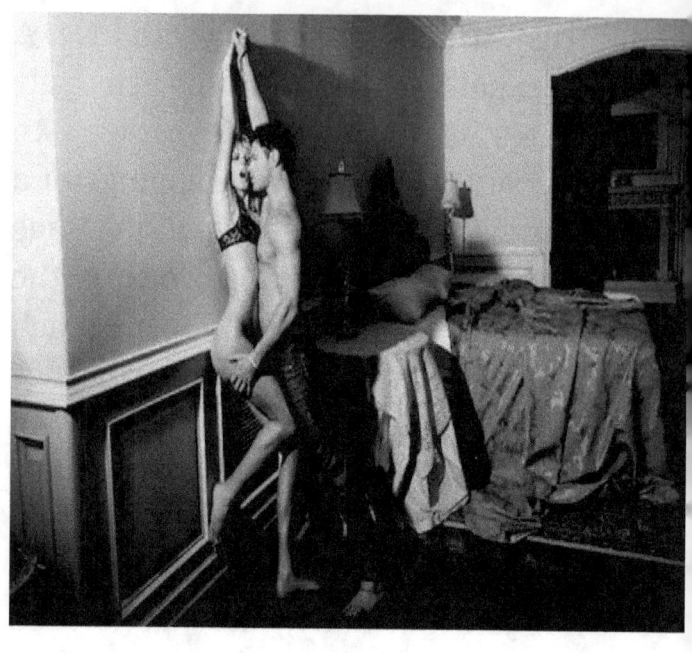

Chapter 2 - The Main Erogenous Zones

How do you do an erotic massage without knowing the body of your partner? The answer is –to study it, millimeter by millimeter. However, so you don't miss the special areas, we have compiled a sample list of places to be sure to stop, because they are proudly called erogenous!

Here they are:

•Shoulders

•Neck

•Thighs (Inner Part)

- Spine

- Chest

- Ears, the surface inside the ears

- Neck, Especially Hairline

- The Skin around the Nipples

- Buttocks

- Popliteal Hole

- Hands, and especially the spaces between the fingers

- The inside of the elbow

- Feet and toes.

Try not to stress during an erotic massage: all this will be felt. Remember your main goal when you give an erotic massage to your loved one – you won't pass an exam on massages. If you ever confuse your movements, it won't be noticed, but if you try to show nerves, your movements will lose smoothness and softness and your partner will notice it immediately.

Do not forget to talk to the man when you give an erotic massage. Of course, not about what you'll be doing this weekend. Tell him how you like how he has just reached your fingertips - his strong arms, his powerful chest or his big penis - choose what you like, and say it with a low voice from the heart.

Be creative and do not be shy.

Chapter 3 - Preparing for Erotic Massage

Atmosphere: Slightly darken the room. You can use candles (preferably with no strong smell), an aroma lamp, or relaxing music. Prepare a place for your lover, making sure it will be comfortable for him to lie and for you to move around him, making your erotic manipulations.

Furniture: A space with a soft covering, 2x3 m. The room should be comfortable, cozy, and the selection of colors must not have an irritating effect, but at the same time attract attention and be warm. The temperature should be 20 - 24 ° C.

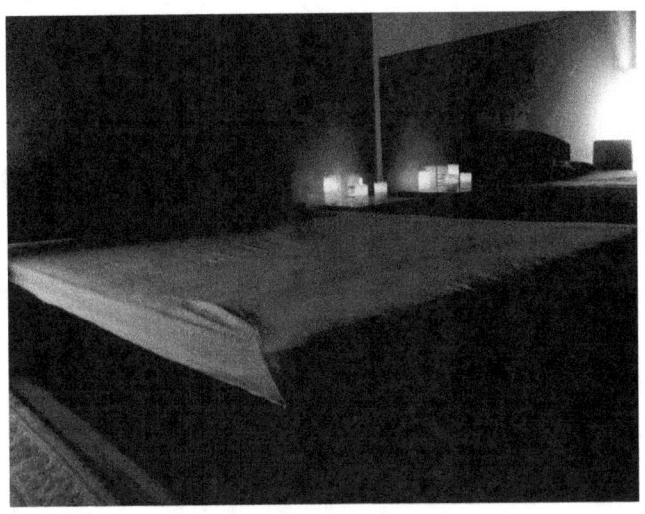

Lighting: It is desirable to have adjustable lighting, candles, etc.

Music: For this purpose you need a special music playlist, in which there are music of various artists— modern, jazz, classical, instrumentals, vocals, popular, nature sounds, meditation, etc. During the massage, put on the music chosen according to the tastes of a partner. You can do without music when silence is desired.

Clothing should be comfortable, erotically cut. For example, for women, comfortable-fit tunics made of natural materials, emphasizing the dignity. And for men - elegant shorts or something like a loincloth, which, incidentally, is suitable for women too. Clothing should be minimal and easily removed. The color of clothing - warm, pleasant, and no annoying tones.

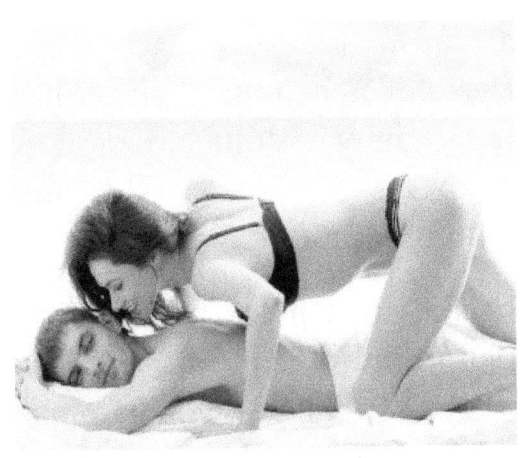

Treats: tea, drinks, and juices. Red Wine - Cahors, brandy in your tea. Fruit, jams, cookies, etc. There should be plenty!!!

Don't let your partner have a heavy meal before the massage. This is extremely important for any massage. But for the erotic massage, it is the most taboo of all taboos; all the energy of the man should be focused on you, rather than digesting a turkey.

To make your partner more relaxed and ready to receive the maximum enjoyment from the massage, while cooking a meal, you can put their wishes into it. For example, think about how you can help the partner to relax and receive an unforgettable experience.

Shower: it is more pleasant for you and him to be clean and fresh as a baby. To do this, you can take a bath together or share a shower; it's bigger and easier to adjust, but then you will need to monitor the degree of excitation for the both of you. Otherwise, you will not get to the massage. In addition, warm water relaxes the body, this will relieve stress and moral and physical tension.

Briefly cut your fingernails. Yes, a big shock for those who like long nails, but if you accidentally touch (and you will touch!) something gentle with your nail, the play is over. Giving an erotic massage means not just stroking;

there are other movements, for which the presence of long nails is undesirable. Moreover, it's frustrating.

Equipment movement in rhythm. During the massage, you should reconcile your breathing—inhaling and exhaling—with the movement of your hand or other body parts, compression, and relaxation, as well as concentrating on the sensations.

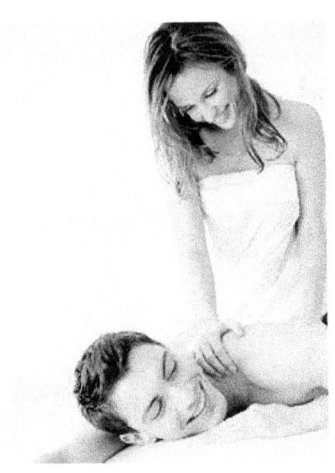

For example, during inhalation, the whole body of the masseuse is relaxed as much as possible, and you massage on exhaling, so you alternate relaxation with tension during the entire massage. This technique allows the massage therapist to keep their power, not get tired of the whole massage, and exercise maximum impact on the partner.

During the massage, there should be nothing on the arms and the body - no jewelry.

It is necessary to concentrate on the movements and sensations.

Fill Sunrik

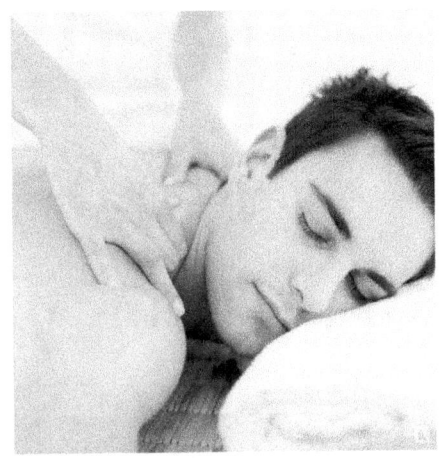

Chapter 4 - Massage for Her

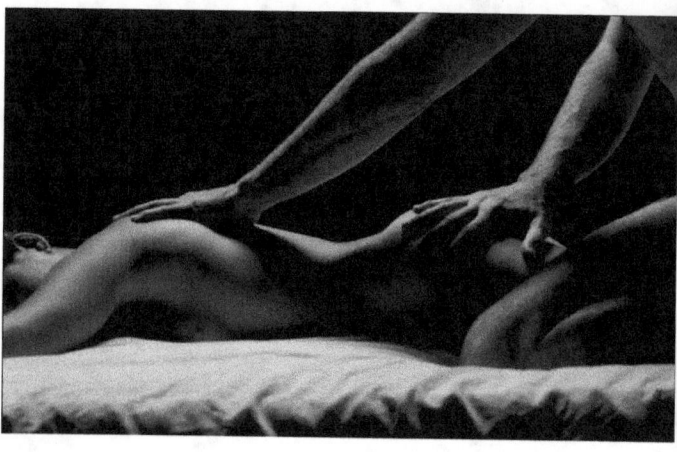

Given the specificity of the female body and psychology, erotic massage, when exposed to the erogenous zones of women, has its own peculiarities. Taking into account that compared to men, women can experience multiple orgasms or protracted, undulating ones during the erotic massage. If a woman on the early stages of massage is ready to reach orgasm, you should not interfere with this. Having the first orgasm, the woman will not lose interest in further erotic massage and will be ready for the next orgasm, because for the majority of women, foreplay is still more important than pure sex. That is, during a single session of erotic massage, woman may experience several orgasms. In contrast to the woman, if the man in the early stages of the erotic massage ejaculates, then, for some men, further steps of the massage are not interesting and even unnecessary.

Erotic massage for women is recommended to start from the upper erogenous zones, gradually descending to the body below the genitals. Directly touching the genitals of women is not recommended, as in this case, the woman is not yet psychophysically totally ready to achieve orgasm. This is due to the action of the hormones - oxytocin affecting uterine contractions. Of course, it is possible without a comprehensive training (only through mechanical stimulation of the genitals of the woman) to bring her to orgasm. But experiencing an orgasm in this way will not give complete satisfaction to a woman because of the gap between the physical and the psycho-emotional sphere. It is known that a woman build up tension more slowly than men, so it takes more time to complete the preparation for sexual release. The recommendations are connected with the fact stated above. It is especially necessary to fulfill or do a clitoris massage. It has already been said that the clitoris has a highly selective sensitivity, and to achieve adequate exposure, you should be very careful and skillful.

We should not forget about the total

psychophysical impact during the erotic massage. This means that, along with the physical effects, the masseuse should work emotionally. That is, a partner should feel that a masseuse is excited, his eyes burning with desire.

Chapter 5 - Massage for Him

You need to determine exactly where you are going to do the massage. Eliminate soft surfaces – if a man is lying on it unevenly, even a gentle massage may cause discomfort. Best suited for the procedure - the floor, lined with soft fabric. If you're going to give him a back massage, put the guy under a rolled towel so as not to disrupt the process of circulation. The situation should be relaxing. Massage can be done both on dry and wet skins. To do this, use a massage lotion.

Easy movement is a massage for hands, feet, neck, and even fingers. It is understood that by staying with your loved ones, you are unlikely to start doing the therapeutic massage against osteoarthritis. But some of the techniques are good. For example, rubbing his hands and feet: do it from the finger to the center of the body. So you'll stimulate lymph flow, making your young man's health only increase. Massaging his body, forget about the rough and sharp movements, take on light and gentle techniques. It may be stroking and rubbing movements or kneading muscles. When the skin is warmed, start vibrating movements of the fingers and the so-called chopping and sawing movements. You need to massage the back, stroking, pinching and gently pulling the skin. The hands and feet give uniform strokes, limbs grasping fingers of his hand like a ring. You can act more vigorously during a massage to the buttocks, as the muscles in this area are protected with large thick skin, so moderate slaps and pinches will be most welcome. All your erotic massage movements will coerce the young man, so do not stop. Massage with lips, stroking his skin with soft tender pieces of fur or silk. A barely perceptible touch better stimulates the sexual impulses of your guy than just rubbing his back. Gently biting his skin, leave the language of small "chain" tracks, carefully write on her fingernails declaration of love. The most sensitive parts of his body - the delicate skin in the crook of the arms and legs, neck, chest, and face. Particularly striking erogenous zones - earlobes, eyelids, and lips. The most delicate part of his body is also impossible to leave without a massage. Be careful; the skin on his manhood is particularly delicate, so I would recommend the light, gentle strokes.

The most important answer to the question of how to do erotic massage for your man is not to be ashamed or shy about anything, do not miss a single centimeter of his body, and to do everything with a sense of movement and desire.

Giving an erotic massage to man, put him on his back. The massage should begin with stroking the chest, and then slowly move to the belly, the inside of the thighs and crotch. Stroking should be for 2 minutes, then pay attention to the testicles; they should be shaken gently and smoothly go ahead for the stimulation of the penis. It is necessary to compress it under the head and massage with hands. On the bottom of the penis in the area where the trunk is connected to the head, the thumb and other fingers should encircle the partner's penis.

The stimulation should be continued until the feeling of approaching ejaculation. In this case, you need to squeeze the head of the penis for 3-4 seconds in order to suppress the ejaculatory reflex. The stimulation can be resumed after about 20-30 seconds. With this, you can control ejaculation and orgasm.

And, of course, if you just take the first steps, it is necessary to observe some rules to avoid ending massage session earlier than you plan to. Your man may reach an orgasm and just go to sleep. Or, on the contrary, he will wait for a long time, but then "biology" will take its course ... and "bye, massage, hello, sex." You were so ready for a massage. This is perhaps the only time when sex can upset, right?

Chapter 6 - Erotic Massage Technique Step By Step

Performing an erotic massage requires some kind of skills, but after reading this section of my book, you can easily master the proper technique. And so...

Erotic massage is a blend of classic massage movements and petting. Classic massage movements are known to many, and we will not stop with them.

Briefly, most massages consist of stroking, kneading, and vibration.

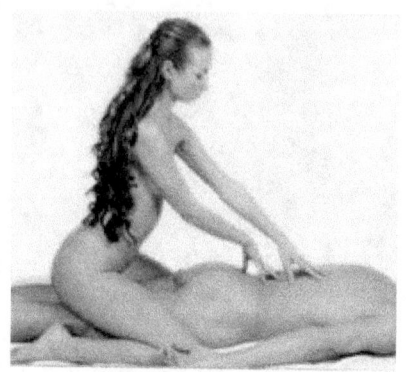

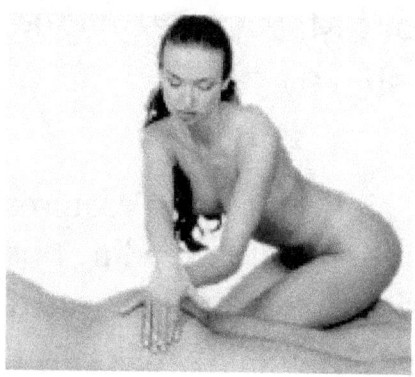

Answering the question of how to do an erotic massage, knowing this, we say that the most important parts - stroking, rubbing - is not as actively performed as in therapeutic massage; your movement scan does not have to be fast, because the shaking will not put your lover in an erotic mood. Kneading is carried out slowly but deeply and accurately. Vibration - it is better to do it the whole hand.

In addition, when giving an erotic massage to a lover, don't repeat any particular technique. Do what you want to do with his body at this moment, as long as you have a clear desire to please him. Some techniques may be absent, being replaced by the language of affection, or something else.

Don't for a second separate your hands from your partner - remember that at least 2 fingers should be touching him; it is felt too energetically.

Start

Start doing better with the erotic massage position "Man lying on his stomach."

Starting with gentle strokes, cajole each

centimeter of partner's body, smooth and heartfelt. Pay attention to your own hands, how relaxed his body under your hands is. Start to relax the whole body.

Massage Rear Surface of the Body

Start with the neck and shoulders, then gently through both hands, go to the lower back and start doing the erotic massage. Then go down with the slight movement of the fingertips and give a hand massage. After that, go to the legs through the buttocks, and massage the legs from the hips to the ankles. A foot massage is better when a partner lies on his back.

During massage of the top of the body, you can sit on a man. The contact of your pubes will definitely have aphrodisiac effects. For foot massage, you still have to get up.

Every movement should go toward the heart, so a back massage begins with the lower back, massage the hands from the hands, foot massage from the ankles. Try massaging the same time, both hands, gently knead each finger. Men love when the skin on the shoulder is grabbed and gently pressed down.

On the back, try to make maximum use of the additional "tools." Help your hands to touch a man with your breasts, teasing him with hot breath.

Hips massage needs to do tricky: massaging thighs touch testicles accidentally. After that, go to the buttocks. Massage movements in this field should be strong. Do not forget the area between the anus and penis. In this area, a massage performed by point movements.

To make even more sensual erotic massage, change the pressure force. Every reception should be performed three times. First - intensive, then weakening, and the third time - barely touching the skin with your fingertips. Strong pressure removes muscle tension. This will help him to relax both physically and emotionally, and increase susceptibility to the more sensual pleasure from the next steps of massage.

Front surface massage

Gently help the man to roll over on his back.

Start doing erotic massage again with the neck and shoulders, moving slowly to the chest and abdomen. Approaching the genitals, as if by chance touch them with the back of the hand or any other body part. And when a man freeze in anticipation of massage, genitals dramatically go to other participants in the body, thereby teasing him.

You can then again begin to massage thighs. During the massage of the hips, do not forget to touch the testicles and the penis itself. When you go to a foot massage, focusing on the inner thighs, which are the erogenous zones. They should all be paid rapt attention -

because you do erotic massage.

When you reach the foot, begin their massage alternately with one hand, while others continue to massage the inner thighs. You can make a foot massage otherwise. With one hand, keep the leg from below the ankle, and the other slowly to rotate the foot. The effect of motion reaches the pelvic and groin muscles and produces an extremely erotic feeling.

Making front erotic massage needs a bit being played; this is the final part of the massage. First, you touch his penis, and then move to the teats, and then returns to the hips and accidentally touch the testicles. In general, you decide, how much to irritate and soothing your man.

All of the above - this is only the movement of the hands. BUT! Do not forget that you still have breath, tongue, lips, hair, and, at the end, his own body. Some of this things must be used during erotic massage! In addition, fingertips perform very erotic movements; just don't tickle a man :) Light biting will please your man, arousing him. You can also use the techniques of holding a feather or tickling the skin with ice cubes.

Erotic massage is designed for long-term holding - two hours or more. It's actually a massage marathon. It consists of several steps:

* Massage in the bath.

* Erotic self-massage.

* Massage dance.

* Massage the soft tissues.

* Erotic massage.

* Therapeutic form of erotic massage

"Bath" or "soap" massage

Fill Sunrik

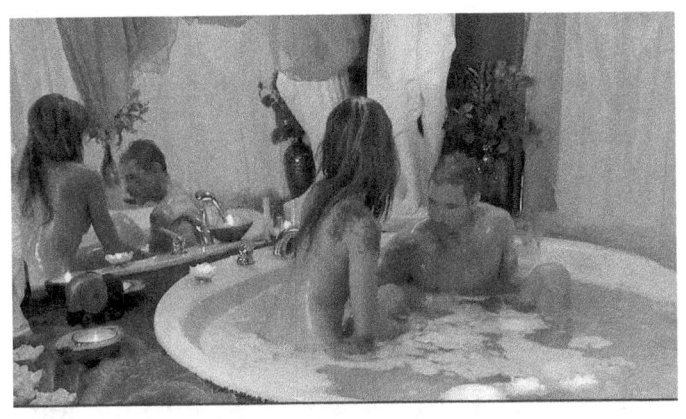

This type of massage can be performed in any adaptation for this purpose place - bath, sauna, pool, etc.

In the extreme case when the appropriate conditions for such a massage is not available, you can use a basin or bucket with warm water - up to 40 ° C.

Prepare a place on the couch or on the floor with a mattress thrown on him.

Top of the mattress cover with plastic wrap or an oilcloth and here spend "soap" massage.

Of course, it should be reserved in advance towels for wiping partner and collect moisture. For soaping the partner, you can use a child or any other soap, mild to the skin.

You can also use special shampoos and gels. The massage is performed with soapy hands or gloves - flannel, fur, etc. Receptions rather superficial - stroking, rubbing, kneading the lungs.

Pre-need to be prepared all the necessary accessories - detergents, clean towels, massage gloves, aromatic oils, etc. Partners should help to undress, carefully remove his clothes and give him bath accessories - bathrobe, slippers, towel, etc. Prepare the water of right temperature, after which you can begin "soap" massage. Soap partner with hands or gloves and begin to massage with above methods. You should not forget, that touches used in principle, it applies not only to the stage of "soap" massage, but also all the other intermediate steps. In this, lies the secret of this - all massage should maintain sexual arousal partner in wave-like shape, that is, something exciting your partner, and then cooling it.

This sexy-sensual contrast is a powerful factor in the activation of hormonal system and human sexual energy generator. After such a contrast "shake" of the body, orgasm at last is strong and bright.

In addition, the hands may be used and other parts of the body: chest, abdomen, buttocks, and others. Touching the partner, change various movements - linear, cross, circle, etc. Soap massage is carried out in different positions: standing, sitting, and lying down - as a good start for the partner and masseur. Time spent on the soap massage, may be about 10-20 minutes. If during the soap massage, the man gets excited and thus, leads to an erection, then it is not recommended to touch his genitals, because this could even increasingly help to bring the man to orgasm. Hence, reduces the interest of men to further stages of erotic massage, and do not give a bright strong satisfaction.

To reduce the excitation of the partner, a level of concentration must be directed to him and to the genital area with a jet of cool water, and apply to the other parts of his body a little more powerful technique. There is a trick: squeeze with fingers, the head of the penis for a few seconds - it promotes blood flow to the head of the penis and reduce sexual arousal.

Once more, during the "soap" massage, it is necessary to monitor the reaction of the partner - at the first sign of his excitement, use the "cooling" means - go for tougher massage techniques such as percussion, to touch the genital area with cool hands, etc.

The air in the room where "soap"

massage is made, can be flavored with scents pleasant for a partner.

After this, massage partner and rinse in the shower or rinse otherwise. Then wipe him dry, harbor bathrobe, and give time to cool down.

Massage in the dance

The next stage - it is a massage in the dance. Of course, it is not necessary, but there are available and known benefits. Firstly, it is a good occasion for further closer contact with a partner. Secondly, the activity contributes to the manifestation of the partner, as in dance, he has the opportunity to work more closely with the masseuse in the physical plane, as well as through the dance to achieve his great looseness and interest in the future program. By the way, a massage in the dance is very good for couples. Perhaps, this is the most convenient and the only type of massage in which both partners can massage each other simultaneously. Married couples that hold mutual massage know that alternately holding massage does not bring pleasure, especially to the one who got the massage first. After the massage, it is a natural desire to stretch the pleasure, relax, but not to start work - to massage your partner. Massage dance does not have this shortage - both partners are free to give pleasure to each other, besides getting both pleasures - dancing.

Before the massage in the dance and after the "bath" should give some respites to the partner. Here, the principle of wave-like sexual longing partner is involved. As mentioned above, it is possible to treat a small amount of alcohol and fruit. Chat a little with him, showing different types of charm. The respite should not be delayed too, and takes about 10-15 minutes. When it is possible to do an erotic self-massage, which gradually turns into a dance massage.

For the massage, dance partner and masseuse should only take a comfortable position in relation to each other. This consciousness is split into three factors: the music, the feeling of partner and rhythmic movements.

For example, consider conventional position in the dance: the girl's hands on the shoulders of the guy and his hands - at the waist or hips of the girl. In this position, for the girl's hands are easily accessible: the shoulders, neck, head and ears of the partner. And for the lips - lips, neck, and chest. Here on these sites, it carries an erotic and exotic massage. For the man's hands: back of a girl, her buttocks, thighs, and lips - those areas around the girl's lips. At the same time, both partners can mutually massaged each other's bodies with their chest and stomach.

After some time, the position of the hands of the partners is reversed. And massage is already going on in other parts of the body. Then, one of the lowers put arm along the body, and the other may be on a shoulder of the partner. The other partner now has free access to half of the body with a lowered down hand and can hold shoulder massage, side of the body and one hand. Then it goes down and the second hand, and lowered - rises, etc. Further, partners may turn their backs to each other and dance, holding each other's hands behind mutually to massage the thighs and buttocks. May be in this situation: one partner is behind the other and face to his back. In this position, his hands can perform massage around the chest, abdomen, and genitals of his partner. And the one who turned his back to the partner can massage his partner's genitals, buttocks, performing a variety of movements. Spaced side gives the possibility to make massage movements on hips and shoulders, etc. That is, you can excel in dance endlessly. Just do not forget that touch should be changeable in all respects: the speed, power, and area of touch. Totality, you should touch the body of the partner in all available places with all the parts, comfortable for massage: hands, lips, tongue, stomach, chest, back, buttocks, thighs, genitals, etc.

Also the dance massage should not bring a partner to orgasm, use cooling touch technique in time, and let your movements become monotonous to sooth the partner. Massage in the dance depends on the willingness of partners and can last up to an hour.

<u>Massage soft tissues</u>

This step comes after the massage and dance designed to reduce arousal after him, and to prepare for a partner erotic massage. To improve the perception of sensations of a partner, you need to relax him as much as possible, to prepare his body and skin to a more subtle and refined sensations. To this end, soft-tissue massage is performed.

In any case, before you start to study techniques of erotic massage, you must first master the techniques of soft tissue massage. It uses the same techniques as in the well-known classical massage. But there are differences. We do massage of the soft tissue in the following order: hands - head - face - neck - back - buttocks - lower limbs - the stomach - the chest. Such a sequence of massage is based on the concepts of Chinese philosophy of Yin and Yang and the circulation of energy in the human body, and others. That is, it is closer to the field of biophysics. The system of massage is based on a physiological basis. Since the initial and determining are still laws of physics, all occurring phenomena such as the biochemical and physiological towards them are secondary. Therefore, the massage should adhere to the following sequence. In modern saying - from electropositive pole - to electronegative pole. This allows to effect on the human body on deeper fundamental levels.

Massage techniques themselves are not something new and are known by masseurs, except the recommendation to adhere to a specific algorithm in the sequence of massage techniques. Remembering this algorithm allows a short time to remember and faster to master the techniques of massage, while also taken into account the physiological effects of massage techniques.

So, here is the sequence of receptions:

1) Stroking

2) Grinding

3) Pulling

4) Kneading

5) Stretching

6) Twisting

7) Vibration

8) Squeezing

9) Pressing

10) Patting

11) Quilting

12) Effleurage

13) Chopping

14) Concussion

15) Felting

16) Shaking

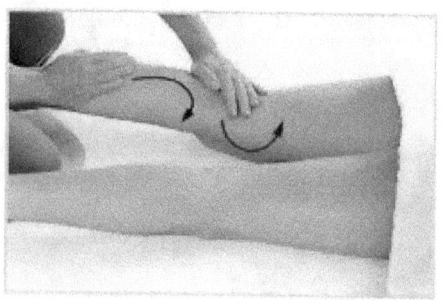

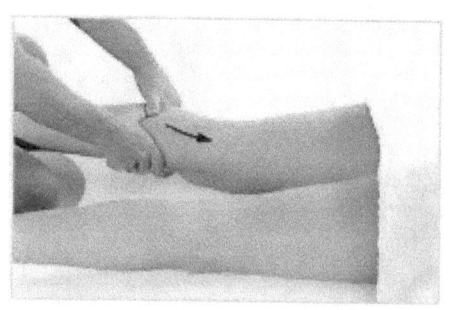

Fill Sunrik

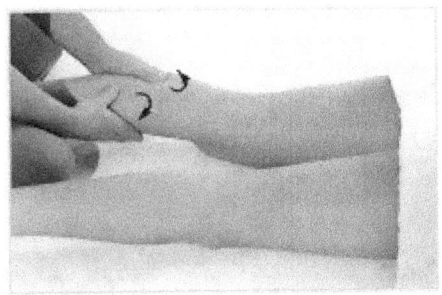

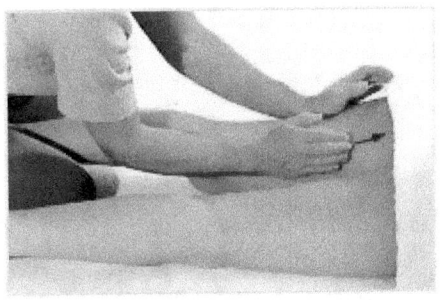

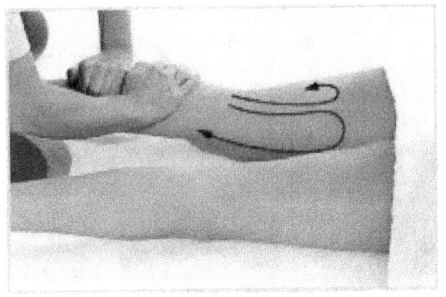

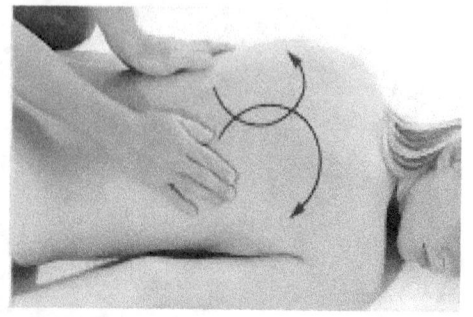

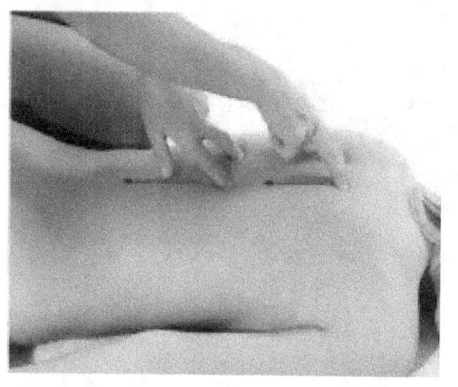

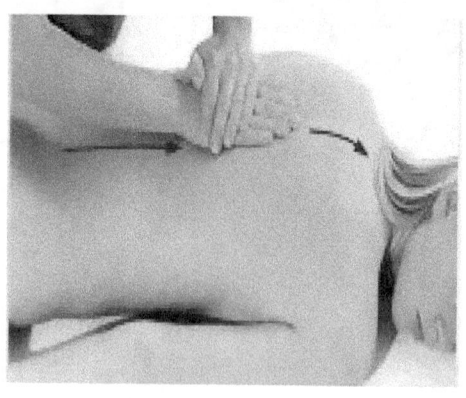

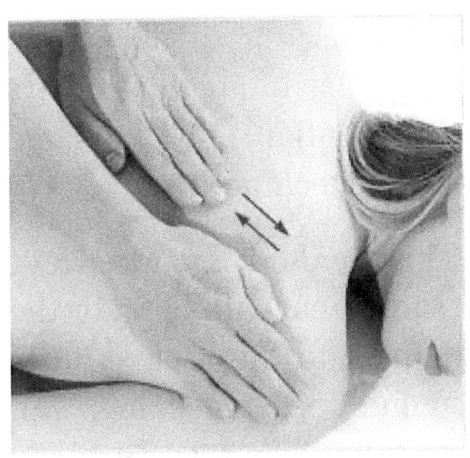

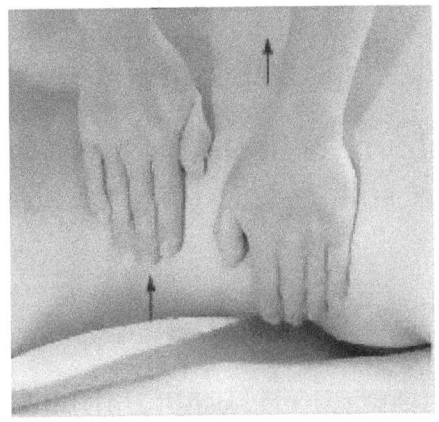

Combinatorial methods: + twisting stretch Vibration + pressing Vibration + squeezing etc.

1. Stroking

This method begins and ends with a massage, it is used among others followed by a reception and the same soft tissue massage techniques.

Technique: This method is carried out gently at the same time with hand or the palm of the hand and the back surface. Hand movements are sweeping, not short. The skin is not displaced. Stroking movements can be linear, transverse, circular, spiral-shaped, zigzag, etc.

It has a calming effect, as well as preparing the soft tissue to a greater impact.

2. Grinding

A stronger reception than stroking carried out with the displacement of the tissue surface of the partner.

Technique: is mainly by palm. Rubbing - energetic, fast, pressing stronger than when stroking. Movement entire, sprawling. Ground to a feeling of warmth, "burning of the skin," until a distinct erythema (redness). It is also possible to carry out grinding with forearm, elbow, and other parts.

It is used to warm up the muscles with myositis, neuralgia, neuritis, and myelitis.

3. Pulling

This technique, as previously mentioned, is carried out after grinding.

Technique: fingers should capture the soft tissue, and pulling them up or to the side, abruptly let go. Thus, both layers of tissue to "tack-free" from each other, which makes them more easily and painlessly displacement relative to each other during subsequent stronger reception.

This technique improves the metabolism in tissues, and acts on the tissue in stimulating way.

4. Kneading

Hold after receiving a pulling.

Technique: fingers grab some tissue and knead it like dough in various directions. The penetration of the fingers into the tissues is the deepest. At the same time, it combines different methods: pulling, squeezing, pressing, stretching, and twisting. Simple kneading can be carried out with palm, palm basis, a fist, elbow, forearm, etc.

It has a strong and comprehensive action on the body.

5. Stretching

Technique: soft tissue is transformed with fingers into the longitudinal cord, and then the cord is stretched longitudinally several times.

It affects the muscles, tendons, nerves, and blood vessels; strengthening them.

6. Twisting

Technique: if the reception is held in the

neck or limbs, the tissue in these areas clasped closely spaced to each other with hands and then make a few movements in opposite directions. Soft tissue between your hands is exposed to twisting.

Reception has an effect on the skin, muscles, tendons, and blood vessels.

7. Vibration

Technique: the reception can be done in different ways - fingertips - this kind of reception is used for acupressure or other portions of the arm: hand, base of the palm, fist, palm edge. At each site, make vibratory action from several seconds to 1-2 minutes.

The reception has a tonic effect on the soft tissues; increases metabolism.

8. Squeezing

Technique: This technique can be performed as the fingers (in the neck, upper and lower limbs, back), and other parts of the hand - palm, edge brushes, fist base of the palm, the whole palm. If the reception is carried out on the limbs, the limbs can be covered with fingers into the ring and push the ring with pressing on the limbs (the direction from the fingertips to the armpits and groin). In other areas, for example, on the back, the tissue can "squeeze" the movement with edge or base of the palm.

A variation of this technique is a method of "roll forward," which is mainly carried out at the back.

Movement held at the same time on the lower back in the upward direction on the back and armpits. The fingers grip the tissue in the form of a roller. The thumbs are located on one side of the roller, and the rest are located in the front row. Thumbs begin to move the roller forward and the other fingers quickly try to catch the tissue, so to the roller is not lost.

Reception improves lymph and blood circulation, has a soothing, relaxing effect.

9. Pressing

Technique: is made by pressing different parts of the arm - the whole palm, base of the palm, fist, finger tips, elbow, forearm, shin, foot, etc.

Admission affects the muscles and blood vessels.

10. Patting

Technique: a few bent palms of the hands. Mainly operate with hands, rather than the entire hand.

Action reception: tones, increases metabolism.

11. Quilting

Technique: made with hand edge. Percussion - transverse from your direction.

Basically, action reception is held on the back, buttocks, and legs.

Action reception: the action tones, increases metabolism.

12. Effleurage

It acts more strongly compared to pat.

Technique: made with different parts of the fist.

Action reception: tones, increases metabolism.

13. Chopping

Technique: alternating strikes caused with edge of the hand

The reception has a tonic effect on the tissue.

14. Concussion

Technique: when performing this technique, any part of the partner's body is covered with a hand or palms of the hands and shaking movements are produced.

For example, if the reception is carried out on the thorax, it has expectorant effect.

Also, the reception has tonic properties.

15. Felting

Technique: This method is used to affect the upper and lower limbs.

Hands of masseuse include muscles of the arms or legs of the partner, and cross-shaking motions are made.

Action reception: the reception has a relaxing nature of the action.

16. Shaking

Massage for Two

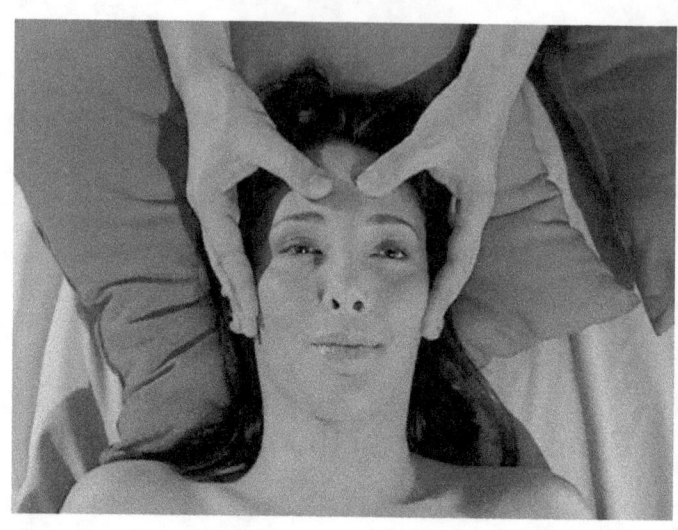

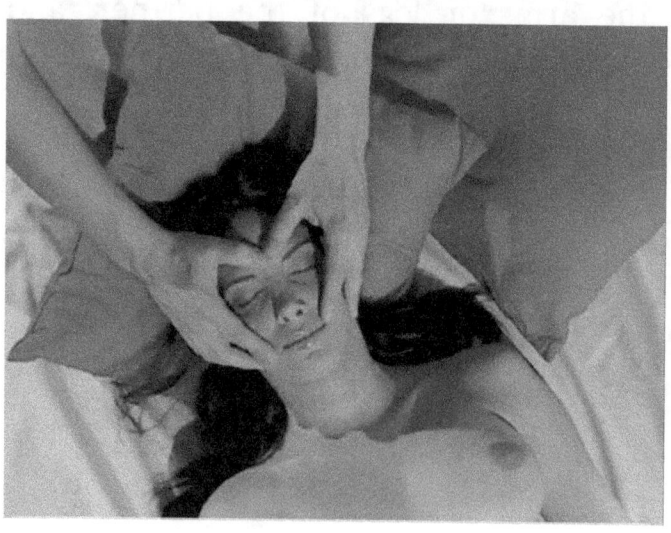

Technique: This technique is primarily used to affect the upper and lower limbs. Hands of masseur cover the foot of the partner, and the therapist makes a few shaking movements.

This method has the relaxing nature of the action.

Let me remind you that these techniques are not limited to the above-mentioned massage techniques, also can be combined with each other, giving a completely new technique.

For example: Vibration + pressing + stretching and twisting, etc.

Massage with heels, toes and soles

It is possible to get both feet on the partner (on the back) and the soles of the feet are made pressing and kneading movements. If the weight of a masseur is more than partner's one, the massage is done with one leg and the other is on the floor.

Toes and the different parts of the foot can be carried out with erotic massage techniques on the partner's genitals and other erogenous zones.

Massage with knee

It is advantageously carried out at the back, spine, sacrum, near the waist, and buttocks.

Massage of the muscles of the hips

Mainly it refers to erotic forms. This massage is performed on the internal surface of the thigh to the buttocks, thighs, and genitals of a partner.

Whole body massage

Basically, a woman-masseuse carried out on a man. Starting position- man lying on his stomach or back. It will be best to grease body with any cream or oil for better sliding. Next, a woman, lying on a man commits a linear, serpentine, circular, lateral movement, touching the entire surface of his body with the body of the partner. That is, by the chest, abdomen, hands, and feet. This method of massage is used in erotic massage.

System rhythmic impact on the partner

This means that their attitude to the partner (physical, emotional, intellectual) should be taken as if the waves swing rhythmically, then with the growth, then decay. What impact does this have on the partner in such particular rhythm? To implement this, it is necessary to determine the temperament of the partner, which is he - melancholic, phlegmatic, choleric, or sanguine. It is known that choleric individuals have the most agile, sharp, and explosive attitudes to situations. They also have a rapid perception. And you should build your physical and emotional relationship more temperamentally, erotic massage movements should be faster in this regard. If they are slow, a partner might not like you to annoy him. On the contrary, melancholics are slow; they have slowed down the perception. Therefore, the therapist should not be more active, than it is required. This applies to emotional and physical communication between them. Since quick massage movements, he simply will not be able to accept them and keep calm. As they say, they should be communicating, "with feeling, plainly, and emphatically." The most harmonious sanguine - desired medium rate handling. Determination of the best speed of massage movements can be empirically. For this purpose, a partner stroking her hand at different speeds, you should ask him to say what the rate of movement is more desirable for it to continue to carry out a massage at a reasonable pace for him.

Chapter 7 - Aromatherapy, Essential Oils to Wake up Feelings

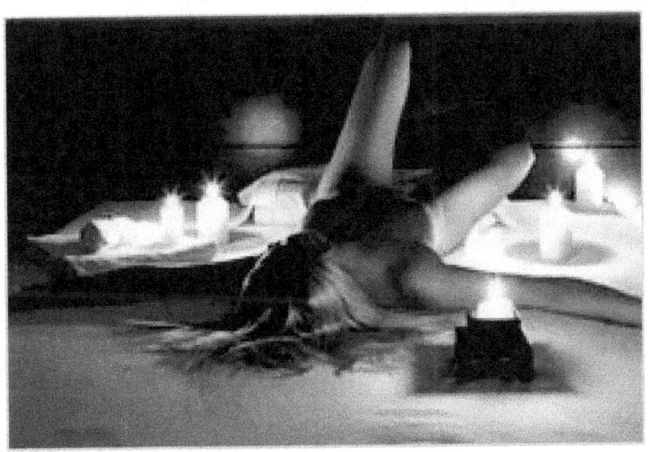

In the tradition of each people are known foods and plants, natural aphrodisiacs - to enhance sexual desire and sexuality. For centuries, people have resorted to odors for erotic games.

The ancient priestesses kept closely

guarded secret recipes for their successful "flavor of love" from the essential oils. Healing art of seduction and using essential oils is more than 5000 years!

Erotic oils - natural aphrodisiacs – were used by well-known lovers. Cleopatra, Nefertiti, Pauline Viardot, Marguerite of Navarre, and Catherine II tested in practice erotic aromatherapy. Legends are composed about their victories and female force.

How useful erotic oils are?

Action, which is provided by natural aphrodisiacs on the body, may be different. This is disinhibiting, removing taboos, stimulating effect, sexuality increasing. And therapeutic effect on the organs of the reproductive system increases the tone of enhancing desire and causing vivid sensations.

These not only excite sensuality, give bright colors, new emotions, but also have great health benefits.

What is the basis of sexual excitement?

Smell! There is nothing strange in the fact that erotic oils aphrodisiacs cause sexual arousal. Sexual behavior and the ability to perceive odors are closely interrelated.

The composition of erotic oils, having aphrodisiacs properties, include pheromones. These ones help attract the attention of others.

Cleverly chosen natural aphrodisiacs, erotic oils, and especially mixtures thereof, awaken erotic associations and set up a body in the desired fashion. Olfactory pulses excite the appropriate emotions, and then affect the genitals.

Well, if there is air ionizer to spray smells into the air. You can also light a special candlesticks or incense. Practice the following method: on a silver platter, located next to the venue of massage sliced, nice smelling fruit, of course, if you do not have allergies. In general, the smell should be selected according to their effect on the psycho-emotional and physical state of the partner, as well as its taste.

Different plants have different effects on the nature of the feelings and the human condition through the so-called essential oils, produced by their special authorities. Aromas plants have healing properties that can relieve fatigue, stress, headaches, lower blood pressure, improve sleep, and much more. This area deals with aromatherapy.

When using essential oils to smell better, make a bottle of oil warm over a candle or a lighter - it promotes faster evaporation of the oil.

It should be noted that the incense should be chosen in connection with the needs of the partner. For example, if he is nervous, irritable, anxious, it is best to spray the smell of lavender as a calming effect, ylang-ylang and sandalwood, the scent of which has a relaxing and antidepressant properties. Also, antidepressant properties have the smell of geraniums, roses, marjoram and sage.

To improve vigor and apathy, use scent of jasmine, rosemary, peppermint, pine, and citrus: bergamot, orange, lemon, mandarin, and others.

The erotic massage in applying some techniques for giving the skin smoothness and flavor of different oils are used.

• Lavender and Rose oil can be used for any skin. To the dry skin - better suited sandalwood, neroli oil and oil clary sage and chamomile.

For oily and acne prone skin to increasingly use cedar, bergamot, cypress, juniper oil. Sandalwood oil is used in frigidity and impotence. Also in the sexual sphere are used oil of rosemary and cedar.

Various oils can be mixed, but should know when to stop and enjoy the taste. When you blend oils skillfully, useful properties of their components are mutually reinforced.

<u>What else is able to affect natural aphrodisiacs - erotic oils?</u>

Anti-aging! Aphrodisiacs have beneficial effects on the skin, smoothing, refreshing it, and giving it elasticity. Active properties provide blood flow to the muscles, awaken sexual energy.

Curative effect! All aphrodisiacs have anti-inflammatory effect, eliminates depression, shy feelings, and uncertainty in your forces. It cannot be lightness and naturalness between lovers; if one feels bad and the other is thinking about work.

Erotic oils optimize blood circulation in the pelvic organs, normalize the work of endocrine and exocrine which in turn increase the cell cycle, and eliminate stagnant processes and decomposition reactions.

With essential oils, natural aphrodisiacs, you will be sexy and full of energy, preserving the health and prolonging the happiest years of sexual life.

What are natural aphrodisiacs for women - the best?

Topping the list of female aphrodisiac sweet and intoxicating scent of the essential oil of **rose**. Rose - exudes tenderness and gives bliss. This aphrodisiac is versatile and suitable for all women and girls, without exception.

Next, an aroma with exciting famous properties - this oil, **ylang-ylang, is** essential - the most powerful natural aphrodisiacs for girls and young women. Slightly bitter smell of flowers - a favorite, not known and expensive perfume.

Seductive and alluring aroma of **neroli**,

essential oil is good where determination and initiative are required. This close to the citrus floral fragrance, is deservedly included in the group of the most exciting aphrodisiac. It refreshes and helps women to overcome shyness.

Bergamot likes those who are short of time. It greatly increases sexual desire. **Geran** helps to relax and do not rush. It is both relaxing and invigorating.

Patchouli and sandalwood oils-create a romantic atmosphere. Their aromas are essential for erotic fantasy and passion awakening.

For true sex gourmets - smells of **jasmine, nutmeg, and cinnamon**. They create an atmosphere of intimacy and luxury.

Why oil mix is better than oil themselves?

Compared with pure essential oils,

aphrodisiacs, a mixture of essential oils has even more pronounced properties. In a mixture, action of oils enhances. They help to increase the potency and sensuality, to extend the love game and physical contact, and also to make sense of the vivid and unique features of the oil mixes.

You can choose a professionally created aphrodisiacs mixes.

Where to buy essential oils, aphrodisiacs?

Get essential oils, cooked by steam distillation, the real, which will not exactly bring you problems.

Watch out for massage oil. In the composition of essential oils, non-natural, are always synthesized chemical components, perfumes and synthetic substrate. The smell of these oils are sharper and noticeably different from those of natural flavors. Essential oils are very expensive, especially aphrodisiacs, because there is always the temptation to dilute them with a chemical analogue.

Some oils aphrodisiacs badly combines with each other, so use one flavor or the final composition that is competently drawn by professionals.

Methods of application of erotic oils, aphrodisiacs

Aromatic components that make up the essential oils - aphrodisiac, enter the body through breathing and skin, getting into the blood and lymph. Depending on what kind of effect is expected from the use of certain essential oils or the selection of the appropriate way in which the natural aphrodisiacs come in our body.

Aroma of erotic range - powerful natural aphrodisiacs. To create an intimate fragrance, **Oil burner** is used in a room, through adding a few drops of oil into the water. Fragrant pair saturates room with light weightless smell and create a romantic atmosphere.

A very good method of flavoring indoor air is **Spraying**. Take the conventional spray, type of water, add 3-5 drops of oil, previously divorced in half a teaspoon of alcohol and spray the room.

Perfect method - **Fumigation** premises erotic oils using a candle or fireplace. Fireplace and candles themselves create the proper atmosphere, and even if we add to this exciting flavor, you will ensure yourself an incredible pleasure.

Put 1-2 drops of oil on the warm candle wax, avoid contact with the wick - essential oils are flammable. There is a fireplace? Sprinkle each piece of wood of the fireplace with three drops of erotic oil composition before ignition of fire. With increasing heat, the aroma will fill the room.

Bed linen and underwear can be flavored by shifting them at the cabinet with paper towels, dropping on them a few drops of essential oils. Vaporized oil will transfer its flavor to underwear.

It is also recommended **to rinse linen** in the water erotic oils or keep in the wardrobe sachet - pads filled with a mixture of aromatic substances - aphrodisiacs.

Aromabaths. How great is to soak together in a warm fragrant bath, enveloping with bliss and charming aromas? There is no spacious bath? No problem! Take a bath with essential oils, aphrodisiacs alone for half an hour before the appointment, and for the mutual joint use erotic massage.

Erotic massage – top of erotic foreplay art. Natural aphrodisiacs - essential oils have special health properties. The aroma of essential oils is erotic and has a very strong psychological impact.

Apply the oil very carefully, just by following the given rules and relationships. A strong smell of oil is able to repel rather than charm.

When applied to the skin, volatile oils and mixtures should be added to the base substrate. Ideal for erotic purposes bearing **avocado oil, pistachios, jojoba, and wheat oils**.

Using the power of erotic oils - natural aphrodisiacs, you will emphasize your natural sexuality, and feel in a completely new way. Essential oils will paint your life with bright colors and will give an extraordinary self-confidence!

Do not be afraid to be more sensual, uninhibited, and frank. Natural aphrodisiacs can help you to overcome the barrier of shyness, give confidence and keep your youth and beauty.

Sometimes, for a full sexual intercourse only need to normalize the person's mental state. Unfortunately, often, a doctor prescribes medicine. In some cases, do not rush to take it. Natural drugs and old folk remedies, including volatile oils, are much smoother and more efficiently.

<u>How to do erotic massage with essential oils?</u>

Areas that should be applied with erotic oil - neck, back of the neck, shoulders, back, rump, feet, and toes.

1. Massage your partner feet and toes with a wide variety of movements - knead, squeeze, pull, bend, and unbend.

2. Stroking back partner from the bottom up along the spine, including the upper part of the buttocks.

3. Rub back in a circular and spiral motion.

4. In the lumbar and sacral areas, use more intensive "sawing" the ribs of palms and rubbing his fist.

5.Massage the shoulders and back of the neck with kneading movements.

6.Finally, spend a few slow circular strokes back, as if spreading the energy throughout the body.

Chapter 8 - Aphrodisiacs Handmade

How to make homemade aphrodisiac?

You want to create your own mix? To prepare aphrodisiacs at home is very easy!

To increase sexual desire. As a basis, use a mixture of natural **vegetable oils of avocado and pistachio** in equal proportions (1: 1)

Take such erotic essential oils:

• The essential oil of rose tree- 15 drops

• Essential oil of ylang-ylang - 15 drops

• Patchouli essential oil - 15 drops

• Essential oil of Indian sandal- 15

drops.

Dilute essential oils in 100 ml of base and use the mixture for an erotic massage, apply the resulting mixture on wet after a shower body and rub until completely absorbed (1 tbsp.) or taking a bath - 20 minutes (after dissolving 1 tbsp. of the mixture in the emulsifier: cream, honey, or salt).

To increase women's sexuality and attractiveness. As a basis, use a mixture of natural vegetable oils **jojoba and wheat germ** in equal proportions (1: 1).

Take such essential oils:

• Geranium essential oil - 15 drops

• neroli essential oil - 15 drops

• Rose essential oil - 10 drops

• Essential oils of verbena - 15 drops.

Dissolve the mixture of essential oils in 100 ml of base and use the mixture for an erotic massage, apply the resulting mixture on wet after a shower body and rub until completely absorbed (1 tbsp.) or taking a bath - 20 minutes (after dissolving 1 tbsp. of the mixture in the emulsifier: cream, honey, or salt).

In order to increase female sensuality. As a basis, use a mixture of natural vegetable oils: **wheat germ and Pistachios** in equal proportions (1: 1).

Take such essential oils:

•Jasmine essential oils   15 drops

•clary sage essential oil   15 drops

•Essential oil of ylang-ylang- 15 drops.

Dissolve the mixture of essential oils in 100 ml of base and use the mixture for an erotic massage, apply the resulting mixture on wet after a shower body and rub until completely absorbed (1 tbsp.) or taking a bath - 20 minutes (after dissolving 1 tbsp. of the mixture in the emulsifier: cream, honey, or salt).

<u>Essential oils handmade</u>. For long-term spread of odors in the room above, as well as for use in erotic massage, you should purchase the appropriate concentrates or oils, or oil is required to cook for themselves. For this, we need to have the right amount of dried plants and some good oil-base: almond, olive, wheat, coconut, or seeds of different plants -sunflower, grape seed, etc.

To prepare the oil with the required properties, taking about 2 tbsp. of dried plants, pour a cup of the oil inside of the above oil that was placed in a dark glass container and placed in a dark place for one month, stored at ambient temperature. The resulting essential oil is added to the base (it can be a more simple oil used for massage, for example, children) in small doses -one drop per teaspoon substrate. One can also add two drops, if it does not cause skin irritation.

Chapter 9 - Aphrodisiacs Meal

Everyone knows that diet greatly affects our lives: what we eat affects our health, weight, state of health ... and not only! Studies show that certain vitamins and minerals increase the production of hormones and thereby stimulate sexual desire. Products-aphrodisiac, which is considered to be the catalysts of passion, should be included in the menu, a romantic dinner for Valentine's Day.

Think about dishes with avocado,

seafood, eggs, celery, bananas, ginger, strawberries, chocolate, honey and garlic, onion (of course, in moderation). I offer a selection of recipes that will make the evening memorable. And turn aphrodisiacs into a daily diet, not just one particular evening!

Aphrodisiacs - these substances and products are able to enhance the amorous passion and ignite the desire in a "chemical" means. Originally, aphrodisiacs were called only plants with exciting properties, and then the products and odors joined this group.

If you think to find an aphrodisiac in "normal" life is not easy, you're wrong. For the "exciting" properties have even the most basic and familiar products, such as eggs or mushrooms. But, of course, champions of their power of love - it's seafood. It does not matter if it's oysters, clams, or shrimp - for a light salad or snack fit all.

Aphrodisiacs at home: food, recipes, tips

Delicious romantic dinner prepared at home, can saturate the body and awaken the sexual hunger. How to achieve this? - Skillfully using aphrodisiac foods (substances that stimulate the libido and sexual activity). If you believe the myths, aphrodisiacs were enjoyed by the goddess of love, Aphrodite. On her behalf, they got their name.

<u>Ordinary products - effective activators</u>

At all times, in different countries used a variety of products- activators, which are conventionally divided into the following groups:

•Fruits and nuts (mangoes, bananas, citrus fruits, figs, apples, avocado, durian, coconut, pine nuts and walnuts, pistachios, peanuts, nutmeg)

•Herbs (ginseng, aloe, angelica)

•Protein and other foods (mushrooms, eggs, red caviar, seafood, olive oil, honey, sesame seeds, sea fish, wheat germ, bee pollen, chocolate)

•Vegetables (onion, seaweed, celery, artichokes, asparagus, carrots)

•Spices and herbs (dill, parsley, coriander, anise, vanilla, cloves, rosemary, curry, ginger, cumin, cinnamon, oregano, basil)

Getting into the male or female body, an aphrodisiac effect on him as well as hormones, thanks to its member pheromones, which increase the potency.

Nutrients and digestible aphrodisiacs act as follows:

• Increase sexual appetite

• Increase the blood flow to the genitals

• Beneficial effect on human hormones

• Increase physical endurance

• Enrich the body "sexual" in vitamin E

• Tone, adds strength

Food of the Gods at home

Food with aphrodisiac is easily made at home. To do this, you need to consider the menu, stock up on necessary food and love to start work. To facilitate the search for food, you can use a selection of original and tested recipes.

Seven of the best erotic salads

Chicken with walnuts

Grind 2 chicken, 3 boiled eggs, a head of lettuce, add 0.5 cups of chopped walnuts, juice of half a lemon, a pack of mayonnaise. Let it brew. Before serving, add the rye crackers.

Fruit

1 pineapple 2 bananas, 4 kiwi cut into slices, mix with 2 tbsp. of chopped nuts and icing sugar, and a pack of vanilla sugar. Pour the fruit syrup and juice of half a lemon.

Of celery root.

Celery root peel, grate. To it, add 1 tbsp. of lemon juice, orange slices, 2 oysters, 3 tbsp. sour cream, salt and sugar to taste.

Avocado salad

2 avocado peeled, cut into cubes, mix with 150 g of cooked shrimp and a jar of canned pineapple, mayonnaise, add spices to taste.

With seaweed.

To add a jar of seaweed boiled egg, chopped onion, grated apple into strips, season with mayonnaise.

With seafood.

140 g squid or shrimp boil in salted water for 5-10 minutes, mixed with 125 g tomatoes, 80 g pickled cucumbers, 140 grams of colored bell peppers, 220 g of Chinese cabbage. Drizzle with oil, lemon juice, soy sauce, pepper. Decorate with seaweed.

Celery and apples.

Grind 100 grams of celery, boiled in salt water, 200 g apples, 200 g of cheese, season with a sauce of vegetable oil and wine.

Romance on the second

Artichokes stuffed with pickled shrimp.

Artichoke clean, boil a little steamed. Prepare the filling: chopped raw shrimp marinated in onions with salt and pepper. Stuff the artichokes and cook for a couple of 45 minutes.

Mushrooms baked with cheese.

400 grams mushrooms clean, cook, separate the legs from the hats. Feet chop, fry. Fry in butter 2 tbsp. flour, dilute the mushroom broth, season with black pepper and salt, mixed with grated cheese. Stuff mushroom caps, baked in the oven.

Veal steak.

The meat, cut into portions and leave for

several hours in a marinade of honey, crushed garlic, ground coriander mixture and pepper, salt, cumin, curry. Then fry on olive oil.

<u>Fish with nuts.</u>

Fillet of sea fish gently discourage, salt and pepper. Dip in beaten egg, then in flour mayonnaise, roll in chopped nuts. Fry in hot oil (preferably olive). Serve cold.

<u>Asparagus cooked.</u>

Young asparagus clear of cuttings, cut into pieces, put in a pan with hot oil, fry over medium heat for 3-5 minutes, add chopped onion, grated carrot, simmer 10 minutes, add salt, pepper, basil, a few spoonfuls of soup, stew the lid further 15 minutes.

Tasty addition to the meal will be a dessert of finely chopped figs filled with blanched almonds and wrapped in coconut, and as a drink, you can use egg liqueur or mulled wine.

Pondering the menu for dinner by candlelight, it is advisable not to overdo it and do not overfeed a partner, so you need to focus on one or two light meals and desserts. It is also important to take into account the concentration of an aphrodisiac, which in too high doses can have the opposite effect. If a woman learns how to use aphrodisiacs skillfully, a couple will create a good mood for a sweet and lasting intimacy.

Chapter 10 - Erotic Self-Massage

If a masseuse does not enjoy the massage, he will not be able to give pleasure through massage to his partner. For example, in the field of sexology known these facts - a higher percentage of women experiencing orgasm until marriage through masturbation, experience orgasms in wedlock also. The percentage of women experiencing an orgasm in sexual intercourse among themselves, but do not cause an orgasm through masturbation before marriage is lesser. Through erotic massage, you should enjoy what he or she does, be excited with a partner and experience the pleasure of his touch. Masseur's excitation through an energy field will also act on the partner, strengthening and stimulating. In addition, the erotic self-massage can be taught to a partner - it will make him more sensitive and responsive to the touch.

Erotic self-massage need to adjust relationship between the partners, it increases the energy of the masseur. This type of massage can be performed on any part of your body, using the technique of "erotic" touch, as described above. Of course, it is especially effective in the erogenous zones and genitals. Erotic self-massage, it is desirable to carry out in a secluded place, where there is good sound insulation. In the extreme case, you can turn an erotic music louder. This is to ensure that during the erotic self-massage, it can be accompanied by different sounds, moans, cries, which contributes to greater build-up of excitement. Erotic self-massage is particularly indicated for persons with reduced excitability, with frigidity and impotence. Erotic self-massage is especially beautiful in dance. This option is good for training partner and it is just recommended to dance massage. Masseuse and partner undress, stand opposite each other and dancing partner repeats the movement of self-massage of erotic masseur. First, erotic exposures are upper area and erogenous zones. Dancing, masseur gently and beautifully holds erotic movements through his hair, ear, neck, lips, and so gradually coming down below - in the chest, abdomen, thighs, buttocks, perineum, and only in the last instance - to the genitals. During this, his body writhing, taking dance erotic poses. During the erotic self-massage partner and a masseuse should feel relaxed and may be accompanied by self-massage erotic dance sighs, moans, and cries. All these, and the very participation of a partner in an erotic self-massage contribute to its more excitement. However, at this stage, he should not be overexcited to such an extent that it ended with an orgasm. This applies mainly to men. For the main program of erotic massage is yet to come, and it may happen that a man gets an orgasm will be enough and further massage program will become uninteresting. And if a woman during an erotic self-massage experiences an orgasm, then it is permissible. In the case of strong excitation, if orgasm is not desirable, it is possible to stop to make a short break, drink a little wine to calm down. Next - or continue erotic self-massage, or go to a steam room massage dance.

Duration of erotic self-massage entirely depends on the attitude and the desire of a partner. On average, you can do an erotic self-massage from 15 to 25 minutes.

Chapter 11 - The Benefits of Erotic Massage

Erotic massage has its philosophical basis and has the following objectives:

1. Self-improving through erotic massage, a massage that is used as a path to self-knowledge and discovering your lover's desires.

2. Achieving the most erotic and sexual satisfaction of your partner.

3. Achieving psychophysical harmony etc.

4. Erotic massage - this is a very important area of human relationships, which can not only solve the problems in the sexual sphere, but also give a lot of fun and pleasure for two.

Chapter 12 - Contraindications to Erotic Massage

They are, in principle, the same as for the classical or therapeutic massage, but less:

* Skin diseases (dermatitis, eczema, etc.), including fungal and pustular.

* Acute respiratory diseases with body temperature above 38 ° C.

* Diseases of the blood capillaries.

* Infectious diseases (the active form of tuberculosis, hepatitis, etc.).

* Sexually transmitted diseases.

* Acute gynecological and urological diseases, etc.

*Acute pain etc.

Chapter 13 - Exotic Erotic Massage

Exotic massage techniques

Massage techniques described below are designed for gourmet experiences. Not all of them are pleasant, but fans may find a variety of feelings among them the most suitable to them. The massage is sometimes not so important in their methods of how the contrast between a variety of sensations and feelings. It is known that the most favorite dish, if it can ever consume, eventually get bored and may even cause disgust.

"Spider"

This first act with two fingers (the little finger and a large) on the body of a partner, then puts the ring, middle, index, and the little finger and thumb break away from the skin and puts closer to the other three, then three fingers moved forward, etc. These movements are reminiscent of an insect crawling on the body.

"Biting of the bird"

All fingers are closed and extended like a beak. Coming together with your fingertips applied carpal rhythmic blows to the body of the partner. Admission is advantageously carried out in the cervical area, on the back, spine and sacrum.

"Tiger Paw"

Fingers of a masseur spread out somewhat bent and stretched. It makes a sharp, wrist capture of the soft tissue partner and then as it comes off the fabric, with a sharp move back, release of tissue. Admission is advantageously carried out on the muscles of the forearm, upper arm, thigh, lower leg, buttocks, that is, the areas where you can capture a tissue. After several seizures, skin reddens and partner "burning."

"Caterpillar"

This puts the base of the palm to any part of the body of the partner, and then straighten the fingers and the palm arc bends backward and the palm surface press the fabric and is rolled on partner's tissue. Then, the base of the palm puts the fingertips, and the movement continues again. Admission is appropriate on the back, legs, male chest.

"Starfish"

Initially, all the fingers of the masseur are collected and put to any part of the body of the partner. Then fingers are disclosed in the form of rays, and break the skin of the partner. Simultaneously with this, the arm moves in a circular motion to the other area of the skin with the fingers start again gradually, at a point, etc. Admission is especially shown at the back, chest, abdomen, buttocks, thighs, neck, and face.

"Swimming fry"

The ribs of both hands of a masseuse sets to any part of the body and by doing hands sharp chaotic movements in different directions, move the hand on the body of the partner, with the bending, then straightening it.

"Snake"

It has two options.

The first option: a partner still standing, sitting or lying down. Masseur with the help of one or two hands on the body slide partner so that it resembles the movement of the snake. These movements can begin with the legs of massaged, gradually moving to the neck and then back. Most importantly, the movement does not stop. To do this, the therapist must be moved around or along a partner and just have time to change his position.

The second option: the therapist may

likely hug a partner while doing wavy arm actions, crouches, then lifts. The partner is between the hands and the body of a masseur and is slowly turned.

Massage, simulates playing musical instruments

"Playing the strings"

At the fingers on the skin of a partner committee movement, reminiscent bust string instruments. This method can be performed on the partner's auricle or on the lateral surface of the body, etc.

"Playing on a drum "

Reminiscent of the effleurage reception in a classic massage. Use different parts of the fist. In terms of the reception of the erotic is more appropriate on the thighs and buttocks.

"Playing the Flute"

Masseur is face to face with a partner, and the fingers of his hands are placed in a row on the spine of the partner, then the fingers are raised, and then lowered to the skin, mimicking playing the flute. The fingers may be positioned on either side of the spine and in a different order. Also, the therapist may be behind a partner and have fingers on his chest. Admission is conveniently carried out in a dance during a massage or standing.

"Playing on the keys"

Masseur's fingers make movements that simulate playing scales. Reception usually runs back, chest, abdomen, buttocks, and genitals of a partner.

Using a variety of objects in an erotic massage

For erotic massage, it is particularly suitable using an exposure of bird's feathers with variety of stiffness. They carried on the erogenous zones, and other parts of the partner's body. Or use fur mittens, gloves, etc. Different kinds of sexual stuff (sold in sex shop) can be used.

Well done, buddy. My congratulations! You have passed a full course of erotic massage art. You were a diligent student! It's time to show your skills to your other half. Come on! Your lover has been waiting for you in your bedroom. Go and surprise him! And your efforts will be appreciated

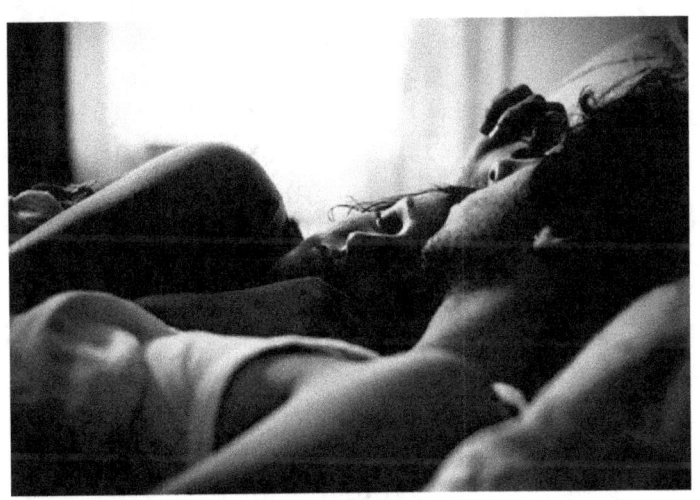

ABOUT THE AUTHOR

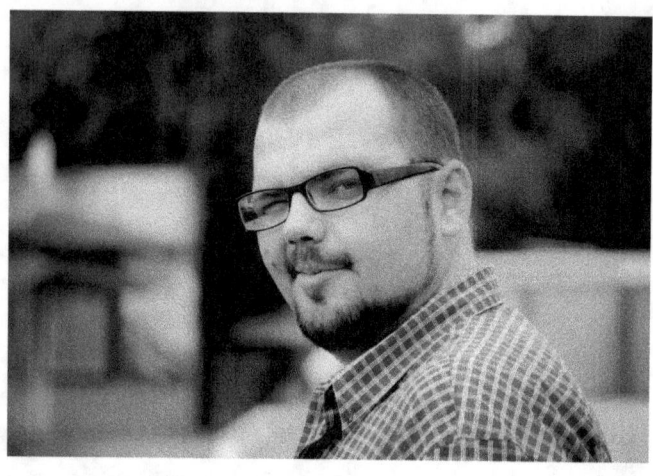

Our life is a fascinating journey and experiment. The more experiments you carry on, the better and more beautiful your life is.
"I love to live, and I write only about the things I'm interested in"
I live in Chicago, Illinois, where I work as a massage therapist and beautician. I have been writing since 30 years, purely it's like a hobby.
My books are based on personal observations and experience, which were got in the process of a personal practical research and experimentation. In my books - the tips provide a detailed

practical information on the issue how to achieve optimal weight, make the skin more healthy and beautiful, look younger, reduce stress levels, strengthen the immune system, to solve many health problems, improve sexual life, thanking to the technique of aromatherapy, massage and self-massage.

My hobbies are: hiking, watching programs on extreme survival, weapon, masterful car driving, self-improvement and self-knowledge. Most of all, I'm enthusiastic about inner harmony and balance, raising self-rating, the science of love to yourself and to the whole world, achievement of success in the chosen field of activity.

I live with my wife and two children in Chicago.

www.ingramcontent.com/pod-product-compliance
Lightning Source LLC
Chambersburg PA
CBHW072103280526
45788CB00006B/2387